Autoimmune Atrophic Gastritis

A Beginner's 3-Step Quick Start Guide to Managing the Condition Through Diet, with Sample Curated Recipes

copyright © 2022 Jeffrey Winzant

All rights reserved No part of this book may be reproduced, or stored in a retrieval system, or transmitted in any form or by any means, electronic, mechanical, photocopying, recording, or otherwise, without express written permission of the publisher.

Disclaimer

By reading this disclaimer, you are accepting the terms of the disclaimer in full. If you disagree with this disclaimer, please do not read the guide.

All of the content within this guide is provided for informational and educational purposes only, and should not be accepted as independent medical or other professional advice. The author is not a doctor, physician, nurse, mental health provider, or registered nutritionist/dietician. Therefore, using and reading this guide does not establish any form of a physician-patient relationship.

Always consult with a physician or another qualified health provider with any issues or questions you might have regarding any sort of medical condition. Do not ever disregard any qualified professional medical advice or delay seeking that advice because of anything you have read in this guide. The information in this guide is not intended to be any sort of medical advice and should not be used in lieu of any medical advice by a licensed and qualified medical professional.

The information in this guide has been compiled from a variety of known sources. However, the author cannot attest to or guarantee the accuracy of each source and thus should not be held liable for any errors or omissions.

You acknowledge that the publisher of this guide will not be held liable for any loss or damage of any kind incurred as a result of this guide or the reliance on any information provided within this guide. You acknowledge and agree that you assume all risk and responsibility for any action you undertake in response to the information in this guide.

Using this guide does not guarantee any particular result (e.g., weight loss or a cure). By reading this guide, you acknowledge that there are no guarantees to any specific outcome or results you can expect.

All product names, diet plans, or names used in this guide are for identification purposes only and are the property of their respective owners. The use of these names does not imply endorsement. All other trademarks cited herein are the property of their respective owners.

Where applicable, this guide is not intended to be a substitute for the original work of this diet plan and is, at most, a supplement to the original work for this diet plan and never a direct substitute. This guide is a personal expression of the facts of that diet plan.

Where applicable, persons shown in the cover images are stock photography models and the publisher has obtained the rights to use the images through license agreements with third-party stock image companies.

Table of Contents

Introduction	7
What Is Autoimmune Atrophic Gastritis?	10
What causes Autoimmune Atrophic Gastritis?	11
What are its symptoms?	12
When to see a doctor?	14
How is it diagnosed?	15
What are the treatments for Autoimmune Atrophic Gastritis?	17
Complications of Autoimmune Atrophic Gastritis	20
Managing Complications	21
Living with Autoimmune Atrophic Gastritis	22
Managing Autoimmune Atrophic Gastritis through Diet and Nutrition	26
Step 1: Prioritize Anti-inflammatory Foods	26
Step 2: Focus on Gut-Healing Foods	29
Step 3: Adapt Your Eating Habits	32
Bonus Tips	34
Foods to Eat and to Avoid	37
Foods to Eat	37
Foods to Avoid	38
7-Day Sample Meal Plan	39
Sample Recipes	43
Baked Flounder	44
Salmon with Avocados and Brussels Sprouts	46
Pecan and Maple Salmon	48
Roasted Broccoli and Salmon	50
Smoked Salmon and Baked Eggs in Avocado	52
Arugula and Mushroom Salad	54
Asparagus and Greens Salad with Tahini and Poppy Seed Dressing	56

Roasted Pumpkin and Brussels sprouts	58
Cauliflower Rice with Chicken and Broccoli	60
Chicken Stir Fry	62
Coconut Milk Berry Pudding	64
Roasted Cauliflower Steaks	66
Sautéed Kale with Garlic	68
Avocado and Spinach Smoothie	70
Conclusion	**72**
FAQ	**75**
References and Helpful Links	**77**

Introduction

Autoimmune atrophic gastritis is a condition in which the body's immune system attacks and destroys the cells lining the stomach. This can lead to a loss of stomach acid and other digestive juices, which can make it difficult to absorb nutrients from food.

Atrophic gastritis involves a scenario where the lining of an individual's stomach undergoes inflammation. This condition tends to develop gradually, spanning several years in many cases.

When the stomach lining is inflamed, it can become thinner and less able to produce stomach acids. This can lead to several health problems, including nutrient deficiencies, ulcers, and an increased risk of stomach cancer.

Atrophic gastritis is most common in older adults, but it can occur at any age. Treatment typically focuses on managing the symptoms and preventing complications. In some cases, surgery may be necessary to remove a portion of the stomach lining that has been damaged by inflammation.

While there is no cure for autoimmune atrophic gastritis, there are treatments that can help manage the condition and improve symptoms. One of the most important things you can do to manage this condition is to eat a healthy diet.

In this quick start guide, we will discuss in detail:

- What causes Autoimmune Atrophic Gastritis?
- What are its symptoms?
- When to see a doctor?
- How is it diagnosed?
- What are the treatments for autoimmune atrophic gastritis?
- Complications of autoimmune atrophic gastritis.
- Risk factors for autoimmune atrophic gastritis.
- Living with autoimmune atrophic gastritis.
- How to manage autoimmune atrophic gastritis through diet and nutrition?

Keep reading as we take a closer look at autoimmune atrophic gastritis, offering insights and guidance on understanding its causes, recognizing symptoms, determining when to seek medical advice, navigating through diagnostic processes, evaluating treatment options, identifying potential complications and risk factors, and adopting effective dietary management strategies.

This guide is designed to empower you with the knowledge needed to manage this condition more effectively, aiming for a proactive approach to health management and an enhanced quality of life.

What Is Autoimmune Atrophic Gastritis?

Autoimmune Atrophic Gastritis is a complex and chronic condition that affects the stomach's lining, leading to significant changes in digestive function. This disorder is characterized by the immune system's misguided attack on the stomach's inner surface, gradually diminishing the stomach cells responsible for producing essential digestive components.

Over time, this autoimmune response results in the thinning or atrophy of the stomach's lining. The progression of this condition can disrupt the stomach's normal operations, impacting the production of stomach acid and intrinsic factors, which are crucial for nutrient absorption. Understanding Autoimmune Atrophic Gastritis is essential for recognizing its impact on gastrointestinal health and overall well-being.

What causes Autoimmune Atrophic Gastritis?

The causes of Autoimmune Atrophic Gastritis center on an autoimmune response where the body's immune system attacks the cells of the stomach lining. This attack leads to the gradual destruction and atrophy of these cells, specifically affecting those responsible for producing gastric acid and intrinsic factors, which are crucial for vitamin B12 absorption. While the exact trigger for this autoimmune response is not completely understood, several key factors are thought to contribute:

1. ***Genetic Factors***: There is evidence to suggest a genetic predisposition to developing Autoimmune Atrophic Gastritis. Individuals with a family history of autoimmune conditions may be at an increased risk.
2. ***Environmental Factors***: Certain environmental triggers, including diet, stress, and possibly bacterial infections (such as with Helicobacter pylori, though more commonly associated with other types of gastritis), might initiate or exacerbate the autoimmune response in genetically susceptible individuals.
3. ***Coexisting Autoimmune Disorders***: The presence of other autoimmune diseases, like Type 1 diabetes, thyroiditis (including Hashimoto's disease), or Addison's disease, may increase the likelihood of developing Autoimmune Atrophic Gastritis,

suggesting a common underlying mechanism of autoimmune dysregulation.
4. *Molecular Mimicry*: This hypothesis posits that the immune system may mistakenly target the stomach lining because it recognizes certain stomach cell proteins as being similar to those of harmful pathogens that the immune system has previously encountered.

These factors illustrate the complexity of Autoimmune Atrophic Gastritis, highlighting the interplay between genetics, environmental exposures, and the immune system in the development of this condition.

What are its symptoms?

The symptoms of Autoimmune atrophic gastritis can vary in severity from person to person. In general, the most common symptoms include:

- *Stomach pain*: Stomach pain is often described as a burning sensation that may radiate to the back or shoulders. In some cases, the pain may be severe enough to interfere with daily activities. If left untreated, atrophic gastritis can lead to ulcers, bleeding, and an increased risk of cancer.
- *Nausea and vomiting*: The most common symptom of autoimmune atrophic gastritis is nausea and vomiting, which can occur after eating even small meals. In some

cases, the vomiting may be so severe that it leads to dehydration and weight loss.
- ***Loss of appetite***: One symptom of autoimmune atrophic gastritis is loss of appetite. This can be a result of the inflammation caused by the disease, as well as the damage to the stomach lining. The symptoms of loss of appetite can vary from person to person and may include feeling full after only a small amount of food or experiencing a lack of hunger altogether. In some cases, loss of appetite can lead to weight loss.
- ***Weight loss***: Weight loss is a common symptom of atrophic gastritis, and it can be caused by several different factors. For instance, the inflammation of the stomach lining can reduce the production of digestive enzymes, which can make it difficult for the body to absorb nutrients from food. People with atrophic gastritis may lose weight due to malabsorption or simple disuse. In severe cases, weight loss can be significant and may require hospitalization.
- ***Feeling bloated***: Or feeling full after eating small amounts of food. One symptom of autoimmune atrophic gastritis is feeling bloated or full after eating small amounts of food. This feeling can be caused by the inflammation of the stomach lining. The inflammation can cause the stomach to produce less acid, which can lead to softer stools and gas. In some

cases, the inflammation can also cause the stomach to produce more acid, which can lead to heartburn.
- ***Heartburn or acid reflux***: Heartburn, also known as acid reflux, is a condition in which stomach acid flows back up into the esophagus. This can cause a burning sensation in the chest and throat.
- ***Burping or gas***: One symptom of autoimmune atrophic gastritis is burping or gas. This occurs when the stomach cannot properly break down food, causing the body to produce excess gas. The gas can cause bloating, pain, and discomfort.

Overall, the symptoms of atrophic gastritis can vary from person to person and may depend on the severity of the condition. It is important to consult a doctor if you experience any of these symptoms to receive proper diagnosis and treatment.

When to see a doctor?

Atrophic gastritis is a condition that occurs when the stomach lining becomes inflamed and starts to thin. This can lead to several symptoms, including indigestion, nausea, appetite loss, and weight loss.

If you experience any of these symptoms, it's important to see your doctor. They can determine if atrophic gastritis is the cause and develop a treatment plan. In some cases, atrophic gastritis can be treated with medication. However, in severe cases, surgery may be necessary to remove damaged tissue. With proper treatment, most people with atrophic gastritis can live normal, healthy lives.

How is it diagnosed?

Atrophic gastritis is a condition that results in inflammation and eventual erosion of the stomach lining. The symptoms of atrophic gastritis can vary depending on the severity of the condition but may include heartburn, indigestion, nausea, and weight loss.

Diagnosing atrophic gastritis can be tricky, as the symptoms are often similar to those of other gastrointestinal disorders. As a result, doctors will often order a combination of tests to rule out other conditions.

Atrophic gastritis is typically diagnosed with one or more of the following tests:

- *Medical History*: As with any diagnosis, your doctor will start by taking a complete medical history. They'll ask about your symptoms and when they started. They'll also ask about your family history of gastrointestinal disorders.
- *Physical Exam*: A physical exam can help your doctor rule out other conditions that may be causing your symptoms. During the exam, they'll likely check your

abdomen for tenderness or other signs of inflammation.
- ***Upper endoscopy***: Upper endoscopy is a procedure where a thin, long tube with a light and camera attached to its end is inserted through the person's mouth and down the throat. The doctor will then be able to see the condition of the person's stomach lining and take a biopsy if necessary.
- ***Biopsy***: During this procedure, a small sample of tissue is taken for further testing. The sample will be looked at under a microscope to see if there are any abnormalities present. The results of the biopsy can help to confirm or rule out a diagnosis of atrophic gastritis.
- ***Blood tests***: Blood tests may be used to determine if a person has atrophic gastritis. Low levels of iron, vitamin B12, or folate can indicate that the body is not able to absorb nutrients properly, which may be a sign of atrophic gastritis.
- ***Stool tests***: In some cases, stool tests may also be ordered to look for evidence of Helicobacter pylori, a bacteria that is known to cause atrophic gastritis.

Atrophic gastritis can often be effectively managed with early diagnosis and treatment. Treatment typically involves a combination of medications, such as proton pump inhibitors or histamine blockers, to reduce stomach acid production.

What are the treatments for Autoimmune Atrophic Gastritis?

While there is no cure for Autoimmune Atrophic Gastritis, a comprehensive treatment plan can significantly help manage the condition and alleviate symptoms. The goal of treatment is to compensate for the body's decreased ability to absorb essential nutrients and to minimize any associated discomforts or potential complications. Here's an overview of the treatment approaches:

1. **Medications**
- *Proton Pump Inhibitors (PPIs)*: These medications reduce the production of stomach acid, which may seem counterintuitive since Autoimmune Atrophic Gastritis leads to reduced acid production. However, they can help in managing symptoms and are particularly useful in cases where there's a need to protect the stomach lining or manage related conditions. Examples include omeprazole (Prilosec), lansoprazole (Prevacid), and pantoprazole (Protonix).
- *Histamine Blockers*: Similar to PPIs, histamine blockers reduce stomach acid production. They target a different pathway by blocking histamine receptors on acid-producing cells in the stomach. Common examples include cimetidine (Tagamet) and ranitidine (Zantac).

- ***Antibiotics***: If an infection, such as Helicobacter pylori, is contributing to the condition or symptoms, antibiotics may be prescribed to clear the infection.

2. **Vitamins and Supplements**

    Given the impaired absorption of nutrients, supplementation is crucial in the management of Autoimmune Atrophic Gastritis:

- ***Vitamin B12***: Essential to prevent or treat pernicious anemia, vitamin B12 supplements are often needed. Given the impaired absorption from the gut, injections or high-dose oral supplements are used.
- ***Iron Supplements***: To combat iron deficiency anemia, iron supplements may be necessary, either orally or, in more severe cases, through IV administration.
- ***Folic Acid***: Supplementation can help address folate deficiency, which is common in individuals with nutrient absorption issues.

3. **Diet**

    A tailored dietary approach is vital for managing Autoimmune Atrophic Gastritis:

- ***Avoiding Trigger Foods***: Identifying and avoiding foods that exacerbate symptoms can help in managing discomfort.

- **_Eating Small, Frequent Meals_**: This can ease the digestive process and reduce symptoms such as bloating and discomfort.
- **_Inclusion of Nutrient-Rich Foods_**: A focus on fruits, vegetables, and whole grains ensures a rich intake of essential vitamins and minerals.
- **_Low-Acid Diet_**: In some cases, a specific diet aimed at reducing acid intake can help manage symptoms.

4. **Surgical Intervention**

   In rare instances where there's significant damage to the stomach lining or the presence of severe complications, surgical intervention may be considered to remove the damaged portion of the stomach.

5. **Monitoring and Follow-up**

   Regular monitoring and follow-up with healthcare providers are essential for managing Autoimmune Atrophic Gastritis. This includes periodic assessments of nutrient levels, surveillance for potential complications, and adjustments to the treatment plan as necessary.

Adopting a comprehensive treatment approach ensures that individuals with Autoimmune Atrophic Gastritis can lead a healthy life, with minimized symptoms and complications. Patients need to work closely with their healthcare team to tailor the treatment plan to their specific needs.

Complications of Autoimmune Atrophic Gastritis

Autoimmune Atrophic Gastritis, characterized by the immune system attacking the stomach's lining, leads to reduced stomach acid production and can result in various complications if not adequately treated. Here is an overview of the potential complications associated with this condition:

Anemia

- *Iron-deficiency anemia*: Due to decreased stomach acid, iron absorption is impaired, leading to a deficiency.
- *Pernicious anemia*: The attack on stomach cells includes those that make intrinsic factors, essential for vitamin B12 absorption, leading to a specific form of anemia characterized by a lack of sufficient healthy red blood cells.

Both forms of anemia associated with Autoimmune Atrophic Gastritis can cause fatigue, weakness, pale skin, and shortness of breath among other symptoms.

Nutrient Deficiencies

The diminished acid environment in the stomach affects the breakdown and absorption of several nutrients, including iron, vitamin B12, folate, calcium, and magnesium. These deficiencies can lead to a range of health issues beyond anemia, such as osteoporosis from calcium and vitamin D malabsorption.

Gastric Cancer

Autoimmune Atrophic Gastritis increases the risk of certain types of gastric cancer, particularly gastric adenocarcinoma and type 1 gastric neuroendocrine tumors. The chronic inflammation and atrophy of the stomach lining create an environment that can lead to the development of malignant cells.

Bleeding and Ulcers

Though less common, the changes in the stomach's environment can lead to an increased risk of ulcers and gastrointestinal bleeding. This complication arises from the damage and inflammation of the stomach lining.

Increased Risk of Infections

A decrease in stomach acid compromises the stomach's ability to act as a barrier to infections. Individuals with Autoimmune Atrophic Gastritis may have an increased risk of intestinal and respiratory infections.

Managing Complications

Recognizing and treating Autoimmune Atrophic Gastritis early is crucial to prevent these complications. Management strategies may include:

- Regular monitoring of blood counts and nutrient levels to identify and treat anemia and nutrient deficiencies early.
- Dietary modifications and supplementation to ensure adequate intake of affected nutrients.
- Periodic endoscopic surveillance to monitor for early signs of gastric cancer or precancerous changes.

Medications, such as proton pump inhibitors or vitamin B12 injections, to manage symptoms and address specific deficiencies.

Consultation with a healthcare provider for regular check-ups and following a tailored treatment plan are vital in managing Autoimmune Atrophic Gastritis and preventing its complications.

Living with Autoimmune Atrophic Gastritis

Living with Autoimmune Atrophic Gastritis requires a comprehensive approach to managing the condition effectively and minimizing the risk of complications. Here are some strategies that can help:

1. **Adhere to Your Treatment Plan**

    Medication Compliance: Follow your prescribed treatment regimen closely, including taking any medications as directed by your healthcare provider. If you experience side effects or have difficulties with your medication, don't hesitate to discuss alternative options with your doctor.

2. **Dietary Considerations**
- *Avoid Trigger Foods*: Identify and steer clear of foods that worsen your symptoms. These can vary from person to person but often include items high in fat, acid, or spices.
- *Small, Frequent Meals*: Eating smaller meals more frequently can help alleviate symptoms by not overwhelming your digestive system.
- *Focus on Nutrient-Rich Foods*: Incorporate a variety of fruits, vegetables, and whole grains into your diet. These foods provide essential vitamins, minerals, and fiber, which are beneficial for overall digestive health.
- *Supplementation*: Based on your doctor's advice, you may need supplements to address specific nutrient deficiencies, such as vitamin B12, iron, calcium, and vitamin D.

3. **Manage Stress**
- *Healthy Stress-Relief Activities*: Engage in activities that reduce stress, such as exercise, meditation, deep-breathing exercises, or yoga. Managing stress can help lessen the symptoms related to Autoimmune Atrophic Gastritis.
- *Seek Support*: Consider joining support groups or seeking counseling if you're struggling to cope with

your diagnosis. Connecting with others who understand what you're going through can be incredibly supportive.

4. **Monitor Symptoms and Communicate with Your Doctor**
- *Regular Monitoring*: Keep a detailed record of your symptoms, dietary habits, and any changes you notice. This information can be invaluable for your healthcare provider in managing your condition.
- *Prompt Reporting of Changes*: Inform your doctor if you notice any new symptoms or if your existing symptoms worsen. Early intervention is key to preventing complications.

5. **Regular Check-ups and Screening**
- *Routine Healthcare Visits*: Regular appointments with your healthcare provider are crucial for monitoring the progression of Autoimmune Atrophic Gastritis and adjusting your treatment plan as needed.
- *Surveillance for Gastric Changes*: Depending on your condition's severity, your doctor may recommend periodic endoscopic examinations to monitor for changes in the stomach lining or early signs of complications.

6. **Lifestyle Adjustments**
- *Quit Smoking*: If you smoke, seek help to quit. Smoking can exacerbate symptoms and increase the risk of complications.
- *Alcohol Moderation*: Limit alcohol consumption, as it can irritate the stomach lining and worsen symptoms.

By actively engaging in your treatment plan, making informed lifestyle choices, and maintaining open communication with your healthcare team, you can manage Autoimmune atrophic gastritis more effectively and sustain a better quality of life despite the challenges of this chronic condition.

Managing Autoimmune Atrophic Gastritis through Diet and Nutrition

Managing Autoimmune Atrophic Gastritis through diet and nutrition involves a comprehensive approach that focuses on mitigating symptoms, preventing nutritional deficiencies, and promoting overall gut health. Here is a three-step guide to effectively manage this condition with diet and nutrition:

Step 1: Prioritize Anti-inflammatory Foods

In managing Autoimmune Atrophic Gastritis, a strategic approach to your diet can significantly mitigate inflammation—a core issue in autoimmune conditions. Prioritizing anti-inflammatory foods is not only pivotal for alleviating symptoms but also for fostering a healthier gut environment. Here's how you can effectively implement this crucial step:

1. Incorporate Omega-3 Fatty Acids

Broaden Your Omega-3 Sources:

While oily fish such as salmon, mackerel, and sardines are well-known for their omega-3 content, don't overlook plant-based sources. Flaxseeds and chia seeds can be easily added to your diet through smoothies, salads, or yogurt.

Walnuts are another excellent source that can be snacked on throughout the day or chopped and sprinkled over dishes for an extra crunch. These healthy fats play a vital role in reducing the body's inflammatory response, offering relief from the discomfort associated with Autoimmune Atrophic Gastritis.

2. Eat a Variety of Fruits and Vegetables

Maximize Antioxidant Intake:

Focus on integrating a rainbow of fruits and vegetables into your meals. Each color represents different antioxidants, which help protect your cells from damage and reduce inflammation.

Dark leafy greens, berries, oranges, and red bell peppers are just a few examples that can boost your vitamin and mineral intake, essential for a robust immune system.

The diversity also ensures you don't miss out on any protective phytonutrients exclusive to certain fruits and vegetables.

3. Choose Whole Grains Over Refined

Fiber for Digestive Health

Substituting refined grains with whole grains like brown rice, quinoa, and oats can have a profound impact on your digestive health. These grains are packed with fiber, which aids in maintaining regular bowel movements and can prevent the constipation often associated with digestive disorders.

Besides their role in supporting a healthy gut flora balance, whole grains are laden with vitamins and minerals that contribute to lowering systemic inflammation. This switch not only helps in managing Autoimmune Atrophic Gastritis symptoms but also supports overall well-being.

By emphasizing these anti-inflammatory food choices, you're not just addressing the immediate discomforts of Autoimmune Atrophic Gastritis; you're also investing in the long-term resilience of your gut health.

Implementing these dietary changes creates a foundation that supports healing and maintenance, reducing flare-ups and improving your quality of life. Remember, dietary adjustments should complement your existing treatment plan, so consult with a healthcare provider before making significant changes to ensure they align with your specific health needs.

Step 2: Focus on Gut-Healing Foods

Focusing on gut-healing foods is an integral step in managing Autoimmune Atrophic Gastritis, as it aids in repairing the stomach lining and enhancing overall digestive health. This approach not only helps in alleviating symptoms but also supports the body's ability to absorb essential nutrients more efficiently.

By incorporating specific types of foods known for their healing properties, individuals can actively contribute to their gut's recovery and maintenance. Here's an expanded overview of how to incorporate these gut-healing foods into your diet:

1. **Bone Broth and Collagen**
- *Healing with Bone Broth:*

   Bone broth is a nutrient-rich liquid made by boiling bones and connective tissues of animals. It is high in collagen, which is instrumental in repairing the damaged gut lining seen in Autoimmune Atrophic Gastritis.

   The amino acids found in bone broth, such as glycine and proline, support the healing of the mucosal lining. Incorporating bone broth into your diet can be as simple as drinking it warm, like tea, or using it as a base for soups and stews.

- *Collagen-Rich Foods:*

    Beyond bone broth, foods like chicken skin, pork skin, fish, and eggs can boost your collagen intake. For vegetarians or those looking for additional sources, a high-quality collagen supplement may also be beneficial. Collagen aids in maintaining the integrity of the gut lining, ensuring a robust barrier against inflammatory triggers.

2. **Fermented Foods for Probiotics**
- *Boosting Gut Flora*: Fermented foods are rich in probiotics, the beneficial bacteria that play a crucial role in maintaining gut health. Regular consumption of yogurt, kefir, sauerkraut, and kimchi introduces a variety of probiotics that can help balance the gut microbiome. This balance is essential for reducing inflammation and improving digestion and nutrient absorption.
- *Incorporation Tips*: Start with small servings of fermented foods and gradually increase the amount to allow your digestive system to adjust. You can add these foods as side dishes, incorporate them into meals, or enjoy them as part of your breakfast or snacks.

3. **Including Prebiotic Foods**
- *Feeding Beneficial Bacteria*: Prebiotic foods contain fibers and natural sugars that feed the beneficial bacteria in your gut. Foods like bananas, garlic, onions, and asparagus are excellent sources of prebiotics. These not only promote a healthy balance of gut flora but also enhance the effectiveness of probiotics.
- *Daily Intake*: Incorporating prebiotic foods into your daily diet ensures that the probiotics in your gut have the necessary nutrients to thrive. These can be easily added to various meals throughout the day, from adding garlic and onions to sauces and soups to enjoying a banana as a healthy snack.

By emphasizing gut-healing foods in your diet, you're taking a proactive step towards managing Autoimmune Atrophic Gastritis and fostering a healthier digestive system. This holistic approach supports the body's natural healing processes, potentially easing symptoms, and contributing to a more comfortable and nutritionally balanced lifestyle.

Remember, while dietary changes can significantly impact gut health, they should complement the medical treatment plan prescribed by your healthcare provider.

Step 3: Adapt Your Eating Habits

Adapting your eating habits is a critical component in managing Autoimmune Atrophic Gastritis effectively. By making mindful choices about not only what you eat but also how and when you eat, you can significantly mitigate the symptoms and improve your overall digestive health. Here's a more detailed exploration of how to implement this crucial step in your daily routine:

1. **Avoid Trigger Foods**
   - *Identify Personal Triggers*: Pay close attention to how your body responds to certain foods. Keeping a food diary can be incredibly helpful in tracking your symptoms to your diet. Note any flare-ups or discomfort following meals and look for patterns.
   - *Eliminate Problematic Foods*: Once you've identified foods that exacerbate your symptoms, work on eliminating them from your diet. Common irritants include spicy foods, which can aggravate the stomach lining; caffeine and alcohol, which can increase stomach acid production; and high-fat foods, which are harder to digest and can slow down the gastrointestinal tract.
2. **Eat Small, Frequent Meals**
   - *Adjust Meal Size and Frequency*: Large meals can overburden your digestive system, leading to increased symptoms. Instead, aim for smaller, more frequent

meals. This approach can help maintain steady energy levels throughout the day and makes it easier for your stomach to digest food.
- *Plan Your Meals*: Try to eat at regular intervals to avoid overwhelming your stomach. Planning can also prevent you from skipping meals or resorting to less healthy options.

3. **Stay Hydrated**
- *Monitor Your Fluid Intake*: Drinking enough fluids is essential for digestion. Water helps break down food, absorb nutrients, and move waste through your intestines. Aim for at least 8 glasses of water per day, adjusting based on your activity level and personal needs.
- *Choose Beverages that Support Digestion*: In addition to water, herbal teas like ginger and peppermint can be soothing for the stomach. Ginger tea can help reduce nausea and inflammation, while peppermint tea may ease digestive discomfort. However, ensure these teas do not conflict with your known triggers or medical advice.

4. **Additional Tips**
- *Mindful Eating Practices*: Pay attention to how you eat, not just what you eat. Eating slowly and chewing thoroughly can aid digestion and nutrient absorption by breaking down food more effectively before it reaches your stomach.

- ***Balance Your Diet***: While focusing on avoiding triggers and eating smaller meals, also ensure your diet remains nutritionally balanced. Incorporate a wide variety of foods to meet your needs for vitamins, minerals, proteins, carbohydrates, and healthy fats.

By adapting your eating habits through these strategies, you can create a supportive environment for your digestive system, alleviating symptoms of Autoimmune Atrophic Gastritis and promoting long-term gut health.

These adjustments, combined with a focus on anti-inflammatory and gut-healing foods, form a comprehensive approach to managing your condition. Always remember to discuss significant dietary changes with your healthcare provider to ensure they align with your overall treatment plan.

Bonus Tips

In managing Autoimmune Atrophic Gastritis, dietary strategy plays a crucial role, but it's essential not to overlook the importance of closely monitoring your nutrient intake and seeking professional guidance for tailored nutritional advice. Here are some bonus tips to further enhance your management plan:

1. **Monitor Your Nutrient Intake**
- ***Stay Vigilant About Nutrient Deficiencies***: Autoimmune Atrophic Gastritis often impairs the stomach's ability to produce enough stomach acid, which is necessary for absorbing certain vitamins and minerals. This can lead to deficiencies in critical nutrients such as vitamin B12, iron, calcium, and vitamin D. These deficiencies not only exacerbate the condition's symptoms but can also give rise to additional health issues if left unaddressed.
- ***Regular Nutrient Level Checks***: Schedule regular appointments with your healthcare provider to test your levels of these key nutrients. Early detection of deficiencies enables prompt intervention, which may include dietary adjustments or supplementation.
- ***Supplementation When Necessary***: Based on your doctor's recommendations, you might need to supplement your diet with specific vitamins or minerals. It's important to follow their guidance on the type and dosage of supplements to avoid over-supplementation, which can carry its own risks.

2. **Consult a Dietitian**
- ***Seek Specialized Nutritional Advice***: Every individual's experience with Autoimmune Atrophic Gastritis is unique, including how it affects their nutritional needs and what triggers they might have. Consulting with a dietitian who specializes in

autoimmune conditions or gastrointestinal disorders can provide you with personalized dietary guidance tailored to your specific situation.

- ***Developing a Customized Eating Plan***: A dietitian can help develop a meal plan that accommodates your nutritional needs while avoiding foods that exacerbate your symptoms. They can also recommend strategies for incorporating anti-inflammatory and gut-healing foods into your diet in ways that suit your tastes and lifestyle.
- ***Navigating Dietary Changes***: A dietitian can be an invaluable resource in helping you understand how to make gradual yet impactful dietary changes, ensuring you do not feel overwhelmed. They can offer practical tips, recipes, and support to help you adjust to your new eating habits.

By integrating these additional strategies into your approach to managing Autoimmune Atrophic Gastritis through diet and nutrition, you can achieve a more comprehensive and effective management plan.

This holistic approach not only aims to reduce symptoms and improve quality of life but also addresses the broader nutritional challenges posed by the condition. Remember, making these changes gradually and under the guidance of healthcare professionals ensures that your dietary adjustments are both beneficial and sustainable in the long term.

Foods to Eat and to Avoid

Managing Autoimmune Atrophic Gastritis through diet involves focusing on foods that are gentle on the digestive system while avoiding those that can cause irritation or exacerbate symptoms. Here is a guide to foods to eat and avoid for individuals following an Autoimmune Atrophic Gastritis diet:

Foods to Eat

These foods are generally considered safe and potentially beneficial for those with Autoimmune Atrophic Gastritis:

- **Lean Proteins**: Skinless poultry, fish, tofu, and lean cuts of meat. These are easier on the stomach and important for maintaining muscle.
- **Low-Fiber Fruits**: Bananas, melons, and cooked fruits can be easier to digest. Avoiding skins and seeds can help as well.
- **Cooked Vegetables**: Gentle cooking methods like steaming or roasting can make vegetables easier to digest. Focus on non-cruciferous options like carrots, spinach, beets, and zucchini.

- *Whole Grains (In Moderation)*: Oats, white rice, and sourdough bread can be included in small amounts. They provide energy without overly taxing digestion.
- *Healthy Fats*: Avocado, olive oil, and coconut oil are good sources of healthy fats that support overall health.
- *Bone Broth*: Rich in nutrients and easy on the digestive system, bone broth can be soothing.
- *Non-Dairy Milk*: Almond milk, coconut milk, and oat milk are lactose-free alternatives to cow's milk.
- *Herbal Teas*: Ginger tea, chamomile tea, and peppermint tea can be soothing for the digestive tract.

Foods to Avoid

These foods may irritate the stomach lining, exacerbate symptoms, or contribute to nutritional deficiencies in individuals with Autoimmune Atrophic Gastritis:

- *High-Fiber Foods*: Whole grains, nuts, seeds, and raw vegetables can be hard to digest for some people.
- *Spicy Foods*: Chili peppers and hot spices may cause discomfort and irritation.
- *Acidic Foods and Beverages*: Citrus fruits, tomatoes, vinegar, and carbonated drinks can aggravate symptoms.

- **High-Fat Foods**: Fried foods, fatty meats, and butter can be difficult to digest and may contribute to discomfort.
- **Dairy Products**: Lactose can be problematic for some people, leading to bloating and discomfort.
- **Processed and Refined Foods**: Processed meats, white bread, pastries, and sugary snacks can contribute to inflammation and offer little nutritional value.
- **Alcohol and Caffeine**: Both can irritate the stomach lining and should be consumed with caution or avoided.
- **Cruciferous Vegetables (for Some)**: While healthy, vegetables like broccoli, cauliflower, and cabbage can cause gas and bloating for some individuals.

It's important to note that dietary tolerances can vary from person to person. Keeping a food diary can help identify specific triggers and guide dietary choices. Consulting with a healthcare provider or a dietitian specializing in autoimmune conditions is recommended to develop a personalized eating plan that meets your nutritional needs and helps manage symptoms effectively.

7-Day Sample Meal Plan

When managing Autoimmune Atrophic Gastritis, it's important to focus on nutrient-dense, anti-inflammatory foods while avoiding triggers that may exacerbate symptoms. Here is a sample meal plan for a week that incorporates these principles:

Day 1

Breakfast: Smoked Salmon and Baked Eggs in Avocado

Lunch: Arugula and Mushroom Salad

Dinner: Chicken Stir Fry

Snack: A handful of mixed nuts (assuming no sensitivity to nuts)

Day 2

Breakfast: Avocado and Spinach Smoothie

Lunch: Roasted Cauliflower Steaks

Dinner: Pecan and Maple Salmon

Snack: Sliced apples with almond butter

Day 3

Breakfast: Coconut Milk Berry Pudding

Lunch: Sautéed Kale with Garlic

Dinner: Cauliflower Rice with Chicken and Broccoli

Snack: Carrot sticks and hummus

Day 4

Breakfast: A bowl of oatmeal topped with sliced bananas and a drizzle of honey

Lunch: Roasted Pumpkin and Brussels sprouts

Dinner: Roasted Broccoli and Salmon

Snack:Greek yogurt with a sprinkle of chia seeds

Day 5

Breakfast: Avocado and Spinach Smoothie

Lunch: Asparagus and Greens Salad with Tahini and Poppy Seed Dressing

Dinner: Baked Flounder

Snack: Fresh fruit salad with a squeeze of lemon (new recipe)

Day 6

Breakfast: Scrambled eggs with spinach and feta cheese

Lunch: Arugula and Mushroom Salad

Dinner: Salmon with Avocados and Brussels Sprouts

Snack: Cottage cheese with pineapple chunks (new recipe)

Day 7

Breakfast: Smoked Salmon and Baked Eggs in Avocado

Lunch: Quinoa salad with cherry tomatoes, cucumber, and feta cheese (new recipe)

Dinner: Cauliflower Rice with Chicken and Broccoli

Snack: A smoothie with banana, kale, and almond milk (new recipe)

Sample Recipes

When managing Autoimmune Atrophic Gastritis through diet, it is important to find recipes that are both nutrient-dense and easy on the digestive system. Here are a few sample recipes that incorporate anti-inflammatory and gut-healing foods recommended for those with this condition:

Baked Flounder

Ingredients:

- 4 flounder fillets (about 1.5 lbs)
- 2 tablespoons extra virgin olive oil
- 1 lemon, zest and juice
- 2 cloves garlic, minced
- 1 teaspoon fresh ginger, grated
- 1 tablespoon fresh parsley, chopped
- 1 tablespoon fresh dill, chopped
- Salt to taste (optional)
- Freshly ground black pepper to taste

Instructions:

1. Preheat Oven: Begin by warming up your oven to 375°F (190°C). Doing so guarantees it's at the perfect temperature for baking the flounder once it's prepped.
2. Prepare the Flounder: Rinse the flounder fillets under cold water and pat them dry with paper towels. This step is crucial for removing any excess moisture that might prevent the fish from baking properly.
3. Season the Fillets: Mix the extra virgin olive oil, zest from a lemon, juice of the lemon, chopped garlic, and shredded ginger in a small bowl. Mix these ingredients well to create a marinade. Brush both sides of each flounder fillet with the marinade, then season with salt (if using) and freshly ground black pepper to taste.

4. Arrange the Fillets: Lay the seasoned flounder fillets in a single layer in a baking dish. Ensure the fillets do not overlap to ensure even cooking.
5. Bake: Place the baking dish in the preheated oven and bake for 10-12 minutes or until the fish flakes easily with a fork. The exact cooking time will depend on the thickness of the fillets, so it's important to check for doneness towards the end of baking.
6. Garnish and Serve: Once baked, remove the flounder from the oven and immediately garnish with fresh parsley and dill. These herbs not only add a burst of flavor but also contribute additional anti-inflammatory benefits.
7. Enjoy: Serve the baked flounder hot, accompanied by a side of steamed vegetables, such as asparagus or green beans, for a complete and nutritious meal.

Salmon with Avocados and Brussels Sprouts

Ingredients:

- 4 salmon fillets (about 6 ounces each)
- 2 tablespoons olive oil
- 1 ripe avocado, sliced
- 1 pound Brussels sprouts, trimmed and halved
- 1 teaspoon garlic powder
- 1/2 lemon, for juice
- Salt to taste (optional)
- Freshly ground black pepper to taste
- Fresh dill or parsley for garnish (optional)

Instructions:

1. Preheat the Oven: Begin by preheating your oven to 400°F (200°C). This ensures the oven is ready for roasting the Brussels sprouts and baking the salmon.
2. Prepare the Brussels Sprouts: Toss the halved Brussels sprouts with 1 tablespoon of olive oil, garlic powder, salt (if using), and black pepper until evenly coated. Spread them out in a single layer on a baking sheet, ensuring they are not overcrowded. Roast in the preheated oven for 20-25 minutes, or until they are tender and the edges are crispy, stirring halfway through the cooking time.
3. Cook the Salmon: While the Brussels sprouts are roasting, prepare the salmon. Brush each salmon fillet

with the remaining olive oil and season with salt (if using) and black pepper. Place the salmon fillets on a separate baking sheet lined with parchment paper for easy cleanup.

4. Bake the Salmon: Put the salmon in the oven and bake for 12-15 minutes, or until the salmon is opaque and flakes easily with a fork. The exact cooking time will depend on the thickness of the fillets.
5. Serve: Once both the salmon and Brussels sprouts are cooked, arrange them on plates. Add slices of ripe avocado to each plate just before serving.
6. Garnish and Enjoy: Squeeze fresh lemon juice over the salmon and avocado for an added zing. Garnish with fresh dill or parsley if desired. The addition of these herbs can enhance the flavor and offer more anti-inflammatory benefits.

Pecan and Maple Salmon

Ingredients:

- 4 salmon fillets (6 ounces each)
- 1/2 cup pecans, finely chopped
- 2 tablespoons pure maple syrup
- 1 tablespoon olive oil
- 1/2 teaspoon garlic powder
- Salt to taste (optional)
- Freshly ground black pepper to taste
- Fresh parsley for garnish (optional)

Instructions:

1. Preheat the Oven: Start by heating your oven to 375°F (190°C). This temperature allows the salmon to cook through while also caramelizing the maple syrup slightly.
2. Prepare the Salmon: Place the salmon fillets on a baking sheet lined with parchment paper. This helps prevent sticking and ensures an easy cleanup.
3. Season the Fillets: In a small bowl, mix the olive oil, maple syrup, garlic powder, salt (if using), and black pepper. Brush this mixture over the top of each salmon fillet, ensuring they are well-coated.
4. Add the Pecans: Sprinkle the finely chopped pecans evenly over the top of each salmon fillet, gently pressing them into the maple syrup mixture to adhere.

5. Bake: Place the prepared salmon in the preheated oven and bake for about 12-15 minutes, or until the salmon is cooked through and flakes easily with a fork. The pecans should be lightly toasted and fragrant.
6. Serve: Carefully remove the salmon from the oven and allow it to rest for a few minutes. This brief resting period lets the juices redistribute throughout the fish, enhancing its natural flavors.
7. Garnish and Enjoy: Transfer the salmon to serving plates. If desired, garnish with fresh parsley for an extra touch of freshness and color. The parsley not only adds flavor but also contributes additional anti-inflammatory benefits.

Roasted Broccoli and Salmon

Ingredients:

- 4 salmon fillets (6 ounces each)
- 1 large head of broccoli, cut into florets
- 2 tablespoons olive oil, divided
- 1 teaspoon garlic powder, divided
- Salt to taste (optional)
- Freshly ground black pepper to taste
- Lemon wedges, for serving

Instructions:

1. Preheat the Oven: Start by preheating your oven to 400°F (200°C), which is an optimal temperature for roasting both salmon and broccoli to perfection.
2. Prepare the Broccoli: In a large bowl, toss the broccoli florets with 1 tablespoon of olive oil, half of the garlic powder, salt (if using), and black pepper until the florets are evenly coated. Spread the broccoli on one-half of a large baking sheet in a single layer.
3. Season the Salmon: Place the salmon fillets on the other half of the baking sheet. Brush each fillet with the remaining olive oil and sprinkle with the rest of the garlic powder, salt (if using), and freshly ground black pepper.
4. Roast: Place the baking sheet in the preheated oven and roast for about 15-20 minutes. The salmon should

flake easily with a fork, and the broccoli should be tender and have crispy edges.
5. Serve: Remove from the oven and transfer the salmon and broccoli to serving plates. Serve immediately with lemon wedges on the side. Squeezing fresh lemon juice over the salmon right before eating adds a vibrant flavor and enhances the absorption of iron from the broccoli.

Smoked Salmon and Baked Eggs in Avocado

Ingredients:

- 2 ripe avocados
- 4 eggs
- 4 slices of smoked salmon
- Salt to taste (optional)
- Freshly ground black pepper to taste
- Fresh dill for garnish
- Lemon wedges, for serving

Instructions:

1. Preheat the Oven: Start by preheating your oven to 425°F (220°C). This high temperature is perfect for baking the eggs inside the avocados.
2. Prepare the Avocados: Cut the avocados in half and remove the pits. Scoop out a bit more flesh from the center to make enough room for an egg in each avocado half. Place the avocado halves in a small baking dish or on a baking sheet to keep them stable while baking.
3. Crack the Eggs: Crack an egg into a small bowl, then gently slide it into the hollowed-out center of an avocado half. Repeat this step with the remaining eggs and avocado halves. It's okay if some of the egg white spills over the edge.

4. Season: Lightly season each filled avocado with salt (if using) and freshly ground black pepper.
5. Bake: Place the baking dish or sheet in the preheated oven and bake for about 15-20 minutes, or until the egg whites are set but the yolks are still runny. You can adjust the cooking time based on how firm you prefer the eggs.
6. Add Smoked Salmon: Once the avocados and eggs are cooked to your liking, remove them from the oven. Immediately top each avocado half with a slice of smoked salmon.
7. Garnish and Serve: Garnish with fresh dill, and serve with lemon wedges on the side. The lemon juice adds a bright flavor and can enhance the absorption of nutrients.

Arugula and Mushroom Salad

Ingredients:

- 4 cups fresh arugula, washed and dried
- 1 cup fresh mushrooms (such as button or cremini), thinly sliced
- 1/4 cup extra virgin olive oil
- 2 tablespoons lemon juice
- 1 teaspoon Dijon mustard (ensure it's mild and suitable for your diet)
- Salt to taste (optional)
- Freshly ground black pepper to taste
- 1/4 cup shaved Parmesan cheese (optional, ensure tolerance)
- Fresh herbs for garnish (e.g., parsley or thyme)

Instructions:

1. Prepare the Dressing: In a small bowl, whisk together the extra virgin olive oil, lemon juice, and Dijon mustard until well combined. Season with salt (if using) and freshly ground black pepper to taste. Adjust the seasoning according to your preference and dietary needs.
2. Slice the Mushrooms: Clean the mushrooms with a damp cloth and slice them thinly. Using fresh mushrooms ensures the salad has a nice, crisp texture and earthy flavor.

3. Toss the Salad: In a large salad bowl, combine the arugula and sliced mushrooms. Drizzle the dressing over the salad and toss gently to coat the leaves and mushrooms evenly. The goal is to lightly dress the salad without overwhelming the delicate flavors of the arugula and mushrooms.
4. Add Cheese: If using, sprinkle the shaved Parmesan cheese over the salad. Parmesan adds a nice depth of flavor and a bit of saltiness, but make sure it's included in your dietary plan before adding it.
5. Serve: Garnish the salad with fresh herbs for an added layer of flavor and a pop of color. Serve immediately to ensure the arugula remains crisp and fresh.

Asparagus and Greens Salad with Tahini and Poppy Seed Dressing

Ingredients:

- 1 bunch of asparagus, tough ends trimmed
- 4 cups mixed salad greens (e.g., spinach, arugula, romaine)
- 1/2 cup shredded carrots
- 1/4 cup tahini (sesame seed paste)
- 2 tablespoons lemon juice
- 1 tablespoon apple cider vinegar
- 1 teaspoon honey (or maple syrup for a vegan option)
- 1 tablespoon poppy seeds
- Salt to taste (optional)
- Freshly ground black pepper to taste
- Water (as needed for consistency)

Instructions:

1. Blanch the Asparagus: Bring a pot of water to a boil. Add the asparagus and cook for 2-3 minutes until they are bright green and tender-crisp. Immediately transfer them to a bowl of ice water to stop the cooking process and preserve their color. Drain and set aside.
2. Prepare the Salad Greens: In a large salad bowl, combine the mixed salad greens and shredded carrots. Toss lightly to distribute the ingredients evenly.

3. Make the Tahini Poppy Seed Dressing: In a small bowl, whisk together the tahini, lemon juice, apple cider vinegar, and honey (or maple syrup) until smooth. If the dressing is too thick, add water, 1 tablespoon at a time, until you reach the desired consistency. Stir in the poppy seeds and season with salt (if using) and freshly ground black pepper to taste.
4. Assemble the Salad: Cut the blanched asparagus into bite-sized pieces and add them to the bowl with the salad greens and carrots. Drizzle the tahini poppy seed dressing over the salad and toss gently to coat everything evenly.
5. Serve: Divide the salad among plates and serve immediately. The freshness of the greens and asparagus paired with the distinctive flavor of the tahini poppy seed dressing makes this salad a delightful, nourishing meal or side dish.

Roasted Pumpkin and Brussels sprouts

Ingredients:

1. 1 small pumpkin (about 2-3 pounds), peeled, seeded, and cut into 1-inch cubes
2. 1 pound Brussels sprouts, trimmed and halved
3. 2 tablespoons olive oil, divided
4. 1 teaspoon dried thyme
5. Salt to taste (optional)
6. Freshly ground black pepper to taste

Instructions:

1. Preheat the Oven: Start by preheating your oven to 400°F (200°C). This temperature is ideal for roasting vegetables, allowing them to become tender inside while caramelizing on the outside.
2. Prepare the Vegetables: On a large baking sheet, spread out the cubed pumpkin. On a separate baking sheet, spread out the halved Brussels sprouts. Drizzle 1 tablespoon of olive oil over each set of vegetables. Toss each set separately to ensure they are well-coated with the oil.
3. Season: Sprinkle the dried thyme, salt (if using), and freshly ground black pepper over both sets of vegetables. Again, toss each set of vegetables to ensure the seasonings are evenly distributed.

4. Roast: Place both baking sheets in the preheated oven. Roast the vegetables for about 25-30 minutes, or until they are tender and start to caramelize around the edges. Halfway through the roasting time, stir the vegetables and rotate the baking sheets to ensure even cooking.
5. Combine and Serve: Once the pumpkin and Brussels sprouts are roasted, combine them in a large serving dish. Toss gently to mix.
6. Optional Garnishes: If desired, you can add a sprinkle of pumpkin seeds or a drizzle of balsamic vinegar before serving for an extra layer of texture and flavor.

Cauliflower Rice with Chicken and Broccoli

Ingredients:

- 1 head of cauliflower, grated or processed into rice-sized pieces
- 2 chicken breasts, boneless and skinless
- 2 cups broccoli florets
- 2 tablespoons olive oil, divided
- 1 teaspoon turmeric
- 1/2 teaspoon garlic powder
- Salt to taste (optional)
- Freshly ground black pepper to taste
- Fresh parsley, chopped for garnish

Instructions:

1. Prepare the Chicken: Start by heating your oven to 375°F (190°C). Season the chicken breasts with half the turmeric, garlic powder, salt (if using), and black pepper. In a skillet over medium heat, heat 1 tablespoon of olive oil. Add the chicken and sear each side for 2-3 minutes until golden brown. Transfer the chicken to a baking dish and bake in the preheated oven for 20-25 minutes, or until the chicken is cooked through and no longer pink inside. Once cooked, remove from the oven, and when cool enough to handle, chop into bite-size pieces.

2. Prepare the Cauliflower Rice: While the chicken is baking, heat the remaining tablespoon of olive oil in a large skillet over medium heat. Add the grated cauliflower, the rest of the turmeric, garlic powder, salt (if using), and black pepper. Cook, stirring occasionally, for 5-7 minutes until the cauliflower is tender. Remove from heat and set aside.
3. Steam the Broccoli: In the meantime, steam the broccoli florets until just tender, about 3-4 minutes. Avoid overcooking to maintain nutrients and a bit of crunch.
4. Combine: Once all components are prepared, add the chopped chicken and steamed broccoli to the skillet with the cauliflower rice. Toss gently to combine over low heat until everything is warmed through.
5. Serve: Garnish with fresh parsley before serving. Enjoy your meal warm.

Chicken Stir Fry

Ingredients:

- 2 boneless, skinless chicken breasts, thinly sliced
- 2 tablespoons olive oil, divided
- 1 cup carrots, julienned
- 1 cup bell peppers (any color), thinly sliced
- 1 cup snow peas
- 1 small zucchini, sliced into half-moons
- 1 tablespoon ginger, minced
- 1 clove garlic, minced (optional, omit if sensitive)
- Salt to taste (optional)
- Freshly ground black pepper to taste

Sauce Ingredients:

- 1/4 cup low-sodium chicken broth
- 1 tablespoon coconut aminos (a soy sauce alternative)
- 1 teaspoon honey (or maple syrup)
- 1 teaspoon arrowroot powder or cornstarch (for thickening)

Instructions:

1. Prepare the Sauce: In a small bowl, whisk together the chicken broth, coconut aminos, honey (or maple syrup), and arrowroot powder until smooth. Set aside.
2. Cook the Chicken: Heat 1 tablespoon of olive oil in a large skillet or wok over medium-high heat. Add the

chicken slices and season with salt (if using) and pepper. Stir-fry until the chicken is cooked through and lightly golden, about 5-6 minutes. Remove the chicken from the skillet and set aside.

3. Stir-Fry the Vegetables: In the same skillet, add the remaining tablespoon of olive oil. Add the ginger (and garlic, if using), stirring quickly for about 30 seconds or until fragrant. Add the carrots, bell peppers, snow peas, and zucchini. Stir-fry for 4-5 minutes until the vegetables are just tender but still crisp.
4. Combine Chicken and Vegetables: Return the cooked chicken to the skillet with the vegetables. Pour the sauce over the chicken and vegetables, tossing well to combine. Cook for an additional 2-3 minutes, stirring constantly, until the sauce thickens and coats the ingredients.
5. Serve: Remove from heat and serve immediately. This dish can be enjoyed on its own or served over a bed of cauliflower rice for a complete meal.

Coconut Milk Berry Pudding

Ingredients:

- 2 cups mixed berries (such as strawberries, blueberries, raspberries, and blackberries), fresh or if frozen, ensure they are thawed
- 1 can (13.5 oz) full-fat coconut milk, ensuring no additives or emulsifiers that may irritate the gut
- 2 tablespoons chia seeds, a great source of omega-3 fatty acids and fiber
- 1 tablespoon honey or maple syrup (optional, depending on dietary restrictions and personal tolerance)
- A pinch of salt (optional, enhances flavor)

Instructions:

1. Berry Puree: In a blender, pulse the mixed berries until you achieve a smooth puree. For a completely smooth pudding, you can strain the puree to remove the seeds, but this step is optional as the seeds contain beneficial fiber.
2. Mix Ingredients: In a large bowl, combine the berry puree with the full-fat coconut milk. Add the chia seeds and mix well. If using honey or maple syrup, and salt, add them at this stage and stir until everything is thoroughly combined.

3. Set the Pudding: Divide the mixture into serving bowls or a large container. Cover and refrigerate for at least 4 hours, or overnight. The chia seeds will absorb the liquid, thickening the mixture into a pudding consistency.
4. Serve: Once set, give the pudding a good stir. It can be served as is or garnished with additional fresh berries on top for extra flavor and a beautiful presentation. A mint leaf can also add a refreshing touch.

Roasted Cauliflower Steaks

Ingredients:

- 1 large head of cauliflower
- 2-3 tablespoons olive oil
- Salt to taste (optional)
- Freshly ground black pepper
- Optional for garnishing: fresh herbs like parsley or thyme

Instructions:

1. Preheat Oven: Begin by preheating your oven to 400°F (200°C). This high temperature is key for achieving a golden, caramelized exterior on the cauliflower steaks.
2. Prepare the Cauliflower: Remove the leaves from the cauliflower and trim the stem without removing too much, as it will help keep the steaks together. Place the cauliflower base down on the cutting board and slice into approximately 3/4-inch thick steaks. Depending on the size of your cauliflower, you should get about 3-4 steaks from one head. Use the remaining florets for another recipe or roast them alongside the steaks.
3. Season: Brush both sides of each cauliflower steak with olive oil. Season with salt (if using) and freshly ground black pepper. The oil not only helps to enhance the flavor but also prevents the steaks from sticking to the baking sheet.

4. Roast: Place the seasoned cauliflower steaks on a large baking sheet in a single layer. Roast in the preheated oven for about 25-30 minutes, or until the edges are crispy and the center is tender. For even roasting, you can gently flip the steaks halfway through the cooking time.
5. Garnish and Serve: Once the cauliflower steaks are roasted to perfection, transfer them to a serving plate. If desired, sprinkle with fresh herbs like parsley or thyme for a burst of flavor and a pop of color.

Sautéed Kale with Garlic

Ingredients:

- 1 bunch of kale, stems removed and leaves roughly chopped
- 2 tablespoons olive oil
- 1-2 cloves of garlic, thinly sliced (optional, can be omitted if garlic is a known irritant)
- Salt to taste (optional)
- A squeeze of fresh lemon juice (for serving)

Instructions:

1. Prepare the Kale: Begin by thoroughly washing the kale leaves to remove any dirt or grit. After removing the tough stems, chop the leaves into bite-sized pieces. Proper preparation ensures the kale cooks evenly and is easier to digest.
2. Heat Olive Oil: In a large skillet or frying pan, heat the olive oil over medium heat. The oil should shimmer slightly when it's ready for the garlic.
3. Sauté Garlic: If using garlic, add the sliced garlic to the hot oil. Sauté for about 30 seconds to 1 minute, just until fragrant. Be careful not to burn the garlic, as this can introduce a bitter taste.
4. Cook the Kale: Add the chopped kale to the skillet. Using tongs or a spatula, stir the kale to coat it with the olive oil and garlic. It may seem like a large amount at

first, but the kale will wilt and reduce in volume as it cooks.
5. Season: Cook the kale for approximately 5-7 minutes, stirring occasionally, until it is wilted and tender. If desired, season with a little salt to taste. Remember, salt should be used sparingly, especially in diets for Autoimmune Atrophic Gastritis.
6. Finish with Lemon: Once the kale is cooked, remove it from the heat. Squeeze a bit of fresh lemon juice over the top before serving. The lemon not only adds a bright flavor but also helps to enhance the absorption of iron from the kale.

Avocado and Spinach Smoothie

Ingredients:

- 1 ripe avocado, peeled and pit removed
- 2 cups fresh spinach leaves, thoroughly washed
- 1 banana, preferably ripe for natural sweetness
- 1 cup unsweetened almond milk (or any other non-dairy milk to avoid dairy-related irritants)
- A small piece of ginger, about 1/2 inch, peeled (optional for added digestive benefits)
- Honey or maple syrup to taste (optional, depending on personal tolerance and dietary restrictions)

Instructions:

1. Prep Your Ingredients: Ensure the avocado and banana are peeled and ready. If you're using ginger, peel it and cut a small piece to avoid overpowering the smoothie.
2. Blend the Greens: Add the spinach leaves to the blender first, followed by the almond milk. Blend these two ingredients until the spinach is completely liquefied. This step ensures there are no leafy chunks in your smoothie.
3. Add the Rest: To the blended spinach and almond milk mixture, add the avocado, banana, and ginger (if using). If you prefer a slightly sweet smoothie, add your chosen sweetener now.

4. Blend Until Smooth: Blend all the ingredients on high speed until the mixture is smooth and creamy. Depending on the power of your blender, this could take anywhere from 30 seconds to a minute. If the smoothie is too thick for your liking, you can add a little more almond milk to reach your desired consistency.
5. Taste and Adjust: Before serving, taste the smoothie. If you feel it needs more sweetness, you can add a bit more honey or maple syrup and blend again.
6. Serve Immediately: Pour the smoothie into glasses and enjoy immediately. For an extra touch of freshness, you can garnish with a few spinach leaves or a slice of avocado.

Conclusion

Congratulations on concluding this in-depth guide on navigating Autoimmune Atrophic Gastritis (AAG) through dietary management. Your commitment to understanding and engaging with this material is commendable and speaks volumes about your dedication to health and well-being. By immersing yourself in the complexities of AAG and the significant role that diet plays in managing this condition, you've taken a substantial step towards empowerment and proactive self-care.

Living with AAG presents unique challenges, especially when it comes to nutrition and diet. However, the insights and strategies discussed throughout this guide are designed to equip you with the knowledge and tools necessary to face these challenges head-on. It's enlightening to discover how certain dietary modifications can not only help manage symptoms but also contribute positively to your overall health.

The guide has underscored the importance of a nutrient-rich diet tailored to meet the specific needs brought on by AAG, including the need for increased vitamin B12, iron, and other essential nutrients that your body might struggle to absorb due to the condition. It highlighted the value of working closely with healthcare professionals to monitor your health and adjust your diet as needed, ensuring that you receive comprehensive support tailored to your unique situation.

Remember, each step you take towards optimizing your diet for AAG management is a step towards a healthier and more comfortable life. This doesn't mean you have to compromise on enjoying food. On the contrary, it opens up a new avenue to explore creative, nutritious, and delicious meal options that cater to your dietary needs while satisfying your palate.

The emphasis on whole foods, lean proteins, fiber-rich fruits and vegetables, and the careful integration of supplements, if necessary, forms a solid foundation for a diet that supports your health without sacrificing enjoyment. It's about making informed choices, understanding the impact of those choices on your body, and finding balance and variety in what you eat.

You're not alone on this journey. Many others are navigating the same path, facing similar challenges, and celebrating shared successes. There's a community out there—a network of support from individuals who understand what you're going through. Engaging with this community can provide additional comfort, motivation, and strategies for managing AAG through diet.

Thank you for taking the time to read through this guide. Your willingness to learn and apply this knowledge to your life is an inspiring testament to your resilience and determination. Managing AAG is a continuous process, one that requires patience, persistence, and a positive mindset. But with the right dietary approach, coupled with regular medical oversight and a supportive network, there is every reason to be optimistic about your ability to lead a fulfilling life despite this condition.

Stay encouraged and continue to advocate for your health with the same zeal you've shown by engaging with this guide. Remember, every day offers a new opportunity to make choices that support your health and well-being. Here's to your continued health, happiness, and success on your journey with AAG.

FAQ

What is autoimmune atrophic gastritis?

Autoimmune atrophic gastritis is a condition in which the body's immune system attacks and destroys the cells lining the stomach. This can lead to a loss of stomach acid and other digestive juices, which can make it difficult to absorb nutrients from food. There is no cure for autoimmune atrophic gastritis, but there are treatments that can help manage the condition and improve symptoms.

What are some common symptoms of autoimmune atrophic gastritis?

Common symptoms of autoimmune atrophic gastritis include indigestion, heartburn, nausea, vomiting, bloating, diarrhea, and weight loss.

What are some common triggers of autoimmune atrophic gastritis?

Several different foods can trigger or aggravate autoimmune atrophic gastritis. It is important to identify which foods trigger your symptoms and avoid them. Some common food triggers include dairy products, wheat, gluten, soy, corn, nightshades (potatoes, tomatoes, peppers, eggplant), citrus fruits, and processed foods.

How can I treat autoimmune atrophic gastritis?

There is no cure for autoimmune atrophic gastritis, but there are treatments that can help manage the condition and improve symptoms. One of the most important things you can do to manage this condition is to eat a healthy diet. You should also avoid trigger foods, supplement your diet with key nutrients, and stay hydrated. If you have severe symptoms, you may also need to take medication to reduce stomach acid production.

How can I prevent autoimmune atrophic gastritis?

There is no known way to prevent autoimmune atrophic gastritis. However, you can reduce your risk by eating a healthy diet, avoiding trigger foods, and supplementing your diet with key nutrients. You should also see your doctor regularly for checkups and get tested for Helicobacter pylori if you are at risk.

How to manage autoimmune atrophic gastritis through diet?

A healthy diet is important for managing autoimmune atrophic gastritis. You should eat plenty of fruits, vegetables, and whole grains. You should also avoid trigger foods, eat small meals, and stay hydrated. Supplementing your diet with key nutrients can also help to reduce symptoms.

References and Helpful Links

Fletcher, J. (2018, June 16). What to know about atrophic gastritis. https://www.medicalnewstoday.com/articles/322153

Vakil, N. (2023, March 8). Overview of gastritis. MSD Manual Professional Edition. https://www.msdmanuals.com/professional/gastrointestinal-disorders/gastritis-and-peptic-ulcer-disease/overview-of-gastritis

Whnp-Bc, L. S. M. B. (2023a, July 26). What are the symptoms of gastritis? https://www.medicalnewstoday.com/articles/307960

What is gastritis? (2024, April 1). WebMD. https://www.webmd.com/digestive-disorders/digestive-diseases-gastritis

Ruscio, & Ruscio. (2024, March 1). What's the best autoimmune atrophic gastritis diet? - Dr. Michael Ruscio, DC. Dr. Michael Ruscio, DC. https://drruscio.com/autoimmune-atrophic-gastritis/

Ruscio, & Ruscio. (2024b, March 1). What's the best autoimmune atrophic gastritis diet? - Dr. Michael Ruscio, DC. Dr. Michael Ruscio, DC. https://drruscio.com/autoimmune-atrophic-gastritis/

Richards, L. (2024, January 15). Foods to eat and avoid on a gastritis diet. https://www.medicalnewstoday.com/articles/gastritis-diet#:~:text=People

%20with%20gastritis%20should%20avoid,on%20the%20type%20and%20cause.

Wells, D. (2024, January 19). What to eat and what to avoid if you have gastritis. Healthline. https://www.healthline.com/health/gastritis-diet

www.ingramcontent.com/pod-product-compliance
Lightning Source LLC
LaVergne TN
LVHW012034060526
838201LV00061B/4608